DR. BARBARA CURE FOR CANCER

The Easy Guide To Healing Cancer Naturally Through Dr. Barbara

O'neil Natural Remedies

Desmond Elias

Table of Contents

COPYRIGHT © 2023

All rights reserved. No part of this publication may be reproduced, distributed, or transmitted in any form or by any means, including photocopying, recording, or other electronic or mechanical methods, without the prior written permission of the publisher, except in the case of brief quotations embodied in critical reviews and certain other noncommercial uses permitted by copyright law.

CHAPTER ONE

Introduction to Dr. Barbara's Herbal Approach to Cancer Treatment

In recent years, there has been a growing interest in complementary and alternative medicine (CAM) approaches to cancer treatment. Among these approaches, herbal medicine has gained attention for its potential to support conventional cancer therapies and improve overall quality of life for patients. One notable figure in this field is Dr. Barbara, whose herbal approach to cancer treatment has garnered significant interest and discussion.

Dr. Barbara's approach is grounded in the principles of holistic medicine, which views health as a balance of physical, emotional, and spiritual well-being. Herbs have been used for centuries in traditional medicine systems such as Ayurveda, Traditional Chinese Medicine (TCM), and Native American healing practices. Dr. Barbara integrates knowledge from these diverse traditions to develop a comprehensive approach to cancer care.

Understanding Cancer and Conventional Treatments

Before delving into Dr. Barbara's herbal approach, it's essential to understand cancer and conventional treatments. Cancer is a complex disease characterized by the uncontrolled growth and spread of abnormal cells in the body. It can arise in various organs and tissues, with different types of cancer exhibiting distinct characteristics and behaviors.

Conventional cancer treatments typically include surgery, chemotherapy, radiation therapy, targeted therapy, and immunotherapy. These treatments aim to remove cancerous cells, shrink tumors, and prevent the spread of cancer to other parts of the body. While these interventions can be effective, they often come with significant side effects and may not address the underlying causes of cancer or support the body's natural healing processes.

The Role of Herbal Medicine in Cancer Treatment

Herbal medicine offers a complementary approach to conventional cancer treatments, focusing on enhancing the body's innate ability to heal and restore balance. Herbs contain bioactive compounds that exert various physiological effects, including anti-inflammatory, antioxidant, immunomodulatory, and anti-cancer properties. When used appropriately, herbal remedies can help alleviate symptoms, reduce treatment-related side effects, and improve overall quality of life for cancer patients.

Dr. Barbara's herbal approach to cancer treatment is based on a deep understanding of the therapeutic properties of medicinal plants and their synergistic interactions within the body. She selects herbs based on their specific actions and targets, tailoring treatment protocols to individual patients' needs and preferences. By combining multiple herbs in carefully formulated preparations, Dr. Barbara aims to maximize therapeutic efficacy while minimizing the risk of adverse effects.

Principles of Dr. Barbara's Herbal Approach

Dr. Barbara's herbal approach is guided by several key principles:

1. **Individualized Treatment**: She recognizes that each patient is unique and requires personalized treatment based on their unique constitution, cancer type, stage of disease, and overall health status. Through thorough assessment and consultation, Dr. Barbara develops customized treatment plans tailored to meet the specific needs and goals of each patient.

2. **Whole-Person Care**: Dr. Barbara takes a holistic view of health, addressing not only the physical aspects of cancer but also the emotional, mental, and spiritual dimensions. She emphasizes the importance of supporting the body's natural healing mechanisms and creating a nurturing environment conducive to overall well-being.

3. **Safety and Efficacy**: Safety is paramount in Dr. Barbara's approach to herbal medicine. She carefully selects high-quality herbs from reputable sources and ensures proper

dosing and administration to minimize the risk of adverse reactions or interactions with other medications. Efficacy is also a priority, and Dr. Barbara continually evaluates treatment outcomes to optimize therapeutic results.

4. **Integration with Conventional Care**: Dr. Barbara's herbal approach is intended to complement, not replace, conventional cancer treatments. She works collaboratively with patients' oncologists and healthcare providers to develop integrated treatment plans that combine the best of both conventional and herbal medicine. This integrative approach aims to enhance treatment effectiveness, minimize side effects, and improve overall outcomes for cancer patients.

Key Herbal Remedies Used by Dr. Barbara

Dr. Barbara employs a wide range of herbal remedies in her cancer treatment protocols, each chosen for its specific therapeutic properties and indications. Some key herbs commonly used include:

1. **Turmeric (Curcuma longa)**: Turmeric is prized for its potent anti-inflammatory and antioxidant properties. It contains curcumin, a bioactive compound that has been studied for its potential anti-cancer effects, including inhibiting tumor growth and metastasis.

2. **Green Tea (Camellia sinensis)**: Green tea is rich in polyphenols, catechins, and other antioxidants that have been shown to have anti-cancer properties. Studies suggest that green tea consumption may help reduce the risk of certain cancers and improve treatment outcomes.

3. **Mushrooms (such as Reishi, Shiitake, and Maitake)**: Certain medicinal mushrooms have immunomodulatory and anti-cancer effects. They contain beta-glucans, polysaccharides, and other bioactive compounds that support immune function and inhibit tumor growth.

4. **Astragalus (Astragalus membranaceus)**: Astragalus is an adaptogenic herb that helps strengthen the immune system and improve resilience to stress. It has been used in traditional Chinese medicine to support cancer patients undergoing chemotherapy and radiation therapy.

5. **Echinacea (Echinacea purpurea)**: Echinacea is known for its immune-enhancing properties and may help reduce the severity and duration of colds and respiratory infections in cancer patients undergoing treatment.

Conclusion

Dr. Barbara's herbal approach to cancer treatment offers a holistic and integrative alternative to conventional therapies. By harnessing the healing power of medicinal plants, she aims to support the body's natural ability to fight cancer, alleviate symptoms, and improve overall quality of life for patients. While further research is needed to fully understand the efficacy and safety of herbal remedies in cancer care, Dr. Barbara's approach represents a promising avenue for exploration and innovation in the field of oncology.

CHAPTER TWO

Understanding Cancer: Causes, Types, and Progression

Cancer is a complex and multifaceted disease characterized by the uncontrolled growth and spread of abnormal cells in the body. It is one of the leading causes of morbidity and mortality worldwide, posing significant challenges to healthcare systems and society as a whole. To effectively combat cancer, it's essential to have a comprehensive understanding of its causes, types, and progression.

Causes of Cancer

Cancer can arise from a combination of genetic, environmental, and lifestyle factors. While the exact cause of cancer is often multifactorial and not fully understood in many cases, several common factors contribute to its development:

1. **Genetic Mutations**: Mutations in specific genes can disrupt normal cellular processes, leading to uncontrolled cell growth and cancer development. These mutations can be inherited from parents or acquired over time due to exposure to carcinogens or other environmental factors.

2. **Environmental Carcinogens**: Exposure to certain environmental factors, such as tobacco smoke, ultraviolet (UV) radiation, ionizing radiation, asbestos, and industrial

chemicals, can increase the risk of cancer development by causing DNA damage and promoting cellular changes.

3. **Lifestyle Choices**: Unhealthy lifestyle habits, such as smoking, excessive alcohol consumption, poor diet, lack of physical activity, and obesity, are significant contributors to cancer risk. These behaviors can promote inflammation, oxidative stress, and hormonal imbalances that fuel cancer growth.

4. **Viral Infections**: Some viral infections, such as human papillomavirus (HPV), hepatitis B virus (HBV), hepatitis C virus (HCV), and Epstein-Barr virus (EBV), have been linked to an increased risk of certain cancers, including cervical, liver, and nasopharyngeal cancer.

5. **Chronic Inflammation**: Prolonged inflammation in the body can create an environment conducive to cancer development by promoting cell proliferation, angiogenesis (formation of new blood vessels), and tissue remodeling. Conditions associated with chronic inflammation, such as inflammatory bowel disease (IBD) and chronic infections, can increase cancer risk.

Types of Cancer

Cancer can affect virtually any part of the body, and there are over 100 different types of cancer identified to date. These cancers are classified based on the tissue or organ of origin, the cell type involved, and the cancer's behavior. Some common types of cancer include:

1. **Carcinomas**: Carcinomas are cancers that originate in the epithelial cells lining the body's internal and external surfaces, such as the skin, lungs, breast, prostate, colon, and pancreas. They account for the majority of cancer cases and are further classified based on their specific location and histological characteristics.

2. **Sarcomas**: Sarcomas arise from the mesenchymal tissues, including bones, muscles, cartilage, and connective tissues. These cancers are less common than carcinomas but can be highly aggressive and difficult to treat.

3. **Leukemias**: Leukemias are cancers of the blood and bone marrow, characterized by the abnormal proliferation of white blood cells (leukocytes). They can be classified into acute or chronic forms based on the rate of disease progression and the type of white blood cells affected.

4. **Lymphomas**: Lymphomas originate in the lymphatic system, which includes lymph nodes, lymphatic vessels, spleen, thymus, and bone marrow. They arise from abnormal lymphocytes (a type of white blood cell) and can be classified as Hodgkin lymphoma or non-Hodgkin lymphoma based on their specific characteristics.

5. **Central Nervous System (CNS) Tumors**: CNS tumors develop in the brain or spinal cord and can be either benign (non-cancerous) or malignant (cancerous). They can arise from glial cells, neurons, or other supporting tissues within the brain and spinal cord.

Progression of Cancer

The progression of cancer involves a series of complex steps, including initiation, promotion, progression, invasion, and metastasis. Understanding these stages is crucial for developing effective prevention strategies and treatment interventions:

1. **Initiation**: Cancer initiation occurs when genetic mutations or other cellular changes disrupt normal growth control mechanisms, leading to the transformation of normal cells into cancerous cells. These initial changes may be triggered by exposure to carcinogens, genetic predisposition, or other factors.

2. **Promotion**: During the promotion stage, cancer cells undergo further genetic and epigenetic alterations that promote their survival, proliferation, and resistance to apoptosis (programmed cell death). Tumor promoters, such as inflammation, hormones, growth factors, and cytokines, play a key role in driving cancer progression during this stage.

3. **Progression**: Cancer progression is characterized by the accumulation of additional genetic mutations and the expansion of malignant cell populations. Tumor cells acquire invasive and metastatic properties, allowing them to invade surrounding tissues, penetrate blood vessels or lymphatic vessels, and spread to distant organs or tissues.

4. **Invasion and Metastasis**: Invasion and metastasis are hallmark features of advanced cancer progression. Cancer cells invade the surrounding tissue through the basement membrane and extracellular matrix, allowing them to access blood vessels or lymphatic vessels. Once in the circulation, cancer cells can travel to distant sites in the body and establish secondary tumors through a process known as metastasis.

5. **Angiogenesis**: Angiogenesis, the formation of new blood vessels, is essential for supplying nutrients and oxygen to growing tumors and facilitating their metastatic spread. Tumor cells release pro-angiogenic factors that stimulate the proliferation and migration of endothelial cells, leading to the formation of new blood vessels within the tumor microenvironment.

In summary, cancer is a complex and heterogeneous disease driven by genetic, environmental, and lifestyle factors. Understanding the causes, types, and progression of cancer is essential for developing effective prevention, early detection, and treatment strategies to combat this devastating disease. Ongoing research efforts aimed at elucidating the molecular mechanisms underlying cancer development and progression are critical for improving patient outcomes and reducing the global burden of cancer.

CHAPTER THREE

Dr. Barbara's Philosophy on Herbal Medicine and Cancer Healing

Dr. Barbara's philosophy on herbal medicine and cancer healing is rooted in a holistic approach that recognizes the interconnectedness of the body, mind, and spirit in the healing process. Drawing upon principles from traditional healing systems, modern science, and her own clinical experience, Dr. Barbara emphasizes the importance of individualized care, whole-person wellness, and the therapeutic potential of medicinal plants in supporting cancer patients on their journey to healing.

Holistic Healing Approach

Central to Dr. Barbara's philosophy is the belief that true healing encompasses more than just the physical aspect of illness. She views health and disease as manifestations of a complex interplay between biological, psychological, social, and spiritual factors. Therefore, her approach to cancer healing goes beyond treating symptoms or eradicating tumors; it seeks to address the underlying imbalances and restore harmony within the body and mind.

Dr. Barbara recognizes that cancer affects not only the physical body but also the emotional and spiritual well-being of patients. She provides compassionate care and creates a supportive environment where patients feel heard, empowered, and valued as active participants in their healing journey. By addressing the emotional and psychological aspects of cancer, Dr. Barbara helps patients navigate the challenges of diagnosis, treatment, and survivorship with resilience and grace.

Individualized Care

Dr. Barbara's approach to herbal medicine and cancer healing is highly individualized, taking into account each patient's unique constitution, cancer type, stage of disease, treatment history, and overall health status. She conducts thorough assessments and consultations to gain insight into patients' specific needs, concerns, and goals for treatment.

Based on this comprehensive evaluation, Dr. Barbara develops customized treatment plans that may include a combination of herbal remedies, dietary recommendations, lifestyle modifications, mind-body practices, and supportive therapies. She tailors her recommendations to address not only the physical manifestations of cancer but also the emotional and spiritual aspects of healing.

Dr. Barbara understands that what works for one patient may not necessarily work for another, and she remains flexible and open-minded in her approach. She encourages patients to actively participate in their care, ask questions, and provide feedback throughout the treatment process. By fostering a collaborative partnership with her patients, Dr. Barbara empowers them to take ownership of their health and make informed decisions about their healing journey.

The Therapeutic Potential of Medicinal Plants

At the heart of Dr. Barbara's approach is the belief in the therapeutic potential of medicinal plants to support cancer healing and promote overall well-being. She draws upon the rich tradition of herbal medicine, incorporating knowledge from diverse cultural healing traditions such as Ayurveda, Traditional Chinese Medicine (TCM), Native American medicine, and Western herbalism.

Medicinal plants contain a myriad of bioactive compounds, including phytochemicals, antioxidants, vitamins, minerals, and essential oils, that exert various physiological effects on the body. Dr. Barbara carefully selects and formulates herbal remedies based on their specific actions and indications, aiming to address the underlying imbalances contributing to cancer while minimizing side effects and toxicity.

Herbal remedies used by Dr. Barbara may include individual herbs or synergistic herbal blends tailored to meet the unique needs of each patient. Commonly used herbs in cancer care may possess anti-inflammatory, antioxidant, immune-modulating, anti-cancer, and adaptogenic properties. Dr. Barbara combines traditional wisdom with scientific evidence to guide her selection and dosing of herbal remedies, ensuring both safety and efficacy in her treatment protocols.

Conclusion

Dr. Barbara's philosophy on herbal medicine and cancer healing embodies a holistic and compassionate approach to care that recognizes the inherent interconnectedness of body, mind, and spirit. By providing individualized care, addressing the root causes of illness, and harnessing the healing power of medicinal plants, she empowers patients to embark on a journey of transformation and self-discovery. Dr. Barbara's philosophy serves as a beacon of hope and inspiration for cancer patients seeking integrative and holistic approaches to healing, nurturing, and restoring balance in their lives.

CHAPTER FOUR

The Role of Nutrition in Supporting Cancer Recovery: Herbal Foods and Supplements

Nutrition plays a critical role in supporting cancer recovery and overall well-being. A balanced diet rich in whole foods, fruits, vegetables, lean proteins, and healthy fats provides essential nutrients that support immune function, promote tissue repair, and reduce inflammation. In addition to conventional dietary recommendations, herbal foods and supplements can complement cancer treatment by providing additional therapeutic benefits. Dr. Barbara recognizes the importance of nutrition in cancer recovery and integrates herbal foods and supplements into her holistic approach to care.

Herbal Foods in Cancer Recovery

Herbal foods are natural sources of bioactive compounds, vitamins, minerals, and antioxidants that can support the body's healing process during cancer recovery. Incorporating a variety of herbal foods into the diet can provide essential nutrients and phytochemicals that promote immune health, reduce inflammation, and support detoxification. Some herbal foods commonly used in cancer recovery include:

1. **Turmeric**: Turmeric is a potent anti-inflammatory herb containing curcumin, a bioactive compound with antioxidant

and anti-cancer properties. Adding turmeric to soups, stews, curries, and smoothies can provide immune-boosting benefits and support overall health during cancer treatment.

2. **Garlic**: Garlic is rich in sulfur compounds, antioxidants, and immune-enhancing nutrients that can support detoxification and promote cardiovascular health. Incorporating garlic into savory dishes, salads, and spreads can help boost immunity and reduce inflammation.

3. **Ginger**: Ginger is known for its anti-nausea, anti-inflammatory, and digestive-supportive properties. Drinking ginger tea or adding fresh ginger to stir-fries, marinades, and smoothies can help alleviate chemotherapy-induced nausea and support gastrointestinal health during cancer treatment.

4. **Cruciferous Vegetables**: Cruciferous vegetables such as broccoli, kale, cabbage, and Brussels sprouts are rich in sulforaphane, indole-3-carbinol, and other phytochemicals with anti-cancer properties. Including cruciferous vegetables in salads, stir-fries, and side dishes can support detoxification and reduce the risk of cancer recurrence.

5. **Berries**: Berries such as blueberries, strawberries, raspberries, and blackberries are packed with antioxidants, vitamins, and fiber that support immune health and reduce oxidative stress. Enjoying fresh berries as a snack, topping

for oatmeal, or ingredient in smoothies can provide anti-inflammatory and anti-cancer benefits.

Incorporating a variety of herbal foods into the diet can enhance nutrient intake, support immune function, and promote overall health during cancer recovery.

Herbal Supplements in Cancer Recovery

In addition to herbal foods, herbal supplements can provide concentrated doses of bioactive compounds and nutrients that support cancer recovery and symptom management. Dr. Barbara may recommend specific herbal supplements based on individual patient needs, treatment protocols, and health goals. Some commonly used herbal supplements in cancer recovery include:

1. **Mushroom Supplements**: Medicinal mushrooms such as Reishi, Shiitake, and Maitake contain beta-glucans, polysaccharides, and other bioactive compounds that support immune function and reduce inflammation. Mushroom supplements are available in various forms, including capsules, powders, and extracts, and can be used to boost immunity and enhance vitality during cancer treatment.

2. **Herbal Extracts**: Herbal extracts such as green tea extract, grape seed extract, and turmeric extract contain concentrated amounts of bioactive compounds with antioxidant, anti-inflammatory, and anti-cancer properties.

These extracts can be used to support immune health, reduce inflammation, and enhance overall well-being during cancer recovery.

3. **Adaptogenic Herbs**: Adaptogenic herbs such as Ashwagandha, Rhodiola, and Holy Basil help the body adapt to stress, regulate cortisol levels, and promote resilience during cancer treatment. Adaptogenic herb supplements can support energy levels, improve mood, and enhance stress management during the challenging phases of cancer recovery.

4. **Probiotics**: Probiotic supplements contain beneficial bacteria that support gastrointestinal health, immune function, and nutrient absorption. Probiotics can help alleviate chemotherapy-induced digestive symptoms such as diarrhea, constipation, and bloating, and promote gut microbiome balance during cancer treatment.

5. **Herbal Antioxidants**: Herbal antioxidants such as Coenzyme Q10, Alpha-lipoic acid, and Resveratrol help neutralize free radicals, reduce oxidative stress, and protect cells from damage during cancer treatment. Herbal antioxidant supplements can support cellular health, enhance detoxification, and reduce the risk of treatment-related side effects.

Before incorporating herbal supplements into their regimen, patients should consult with a qualified healthcare provider, preferably one knowledgeable in integrative oncology, to ensure safety, appropriateness, and compatibility with existing treatment protocols.

Conclusion

In conclusion, herbal foods and supplements can play a valuable role in supporting cancer recovery by providing essential nutrients, phytochemicals, and bioactive compounds that promote immune health, reduce inflammation, and support overall well-being. Dr. Barbara recognizes the importance of nutrition in cancer care and integrates herbal foods and supplements into her holistic approach to support patients on their healing journey. By incorporating a variety of herbal foods and supplements into the diet, patients can enhance their nutrient intake, alleviate treatment-related symptoms, and optimize their quality of life during cancer recovery.

CHAPTER FIVE

Key Herbs and Plants for Cancer Treatment and Symptom Management

Herbs and plants have been used for centuries in traditional medicine systems to support health and well-being, including in the context of cancer treatment and symptom management. While herbal medicine should be used as a complementary approach alongside conventional cancer therapies, certain herbs and plants have shown promise in supporting cancer treatment, alleviating treatment-related symptoms, and improving overall quality of life for patients. Dr. Barbara incorporates a variety of key herbs and plants into her holistic approach to cancer care, selecting them based on their specific therapeutic properties and indications.

Turmeric (Curcuma longa)

Turmeric is one of the most extensively studied herbs for its potential anti-cancer properties. It contains curcumin, a bioactive compound with powerful antioxidant, anti-inflammatory, and anti-cancer effects. Curcumin has been shown to inhibit cancer cell proliferation, induce apoptosis (programmed cell death), suppress tumor growth and metastasis, and enhance the efficacy of conventional cancer therapies. Turmeric can be consumed fresh, dried, or in powdered form and incorporated into various dishes, teas, smoothies, and supplements.

Green Tea (Camellia sinensis)

Green tea is rich in polyphenols, catechins, and other antioxidants that have been studied for their anti-cancer effects. Epigallocatechin gallate (EGCG), the most abundant catechin in green tea, has been shown to inhibit tumor growth, angiogenesis (formation of new blood vessels), and metastasis, and induce apoptosis in cancer cells. Green tea consumption has been associated with a reduced risk of several cancers, including breast, prostate, lung, and colorectal cancer. Green tea can be enjoyed as a beverage or taken as a supplement.

Reishi Mushroom (Ganoderma lucidum)

Reishi mushroom, also known as Lingzhi in Traditional Chinese Medicine (TCM), is revered for its immune-modulating, anti-inflammatory, and anti-cancer properties. Reishi contains bioactive compounds such as polysaccharides, triterpenes, and ganoderic acids that support immune function, reduce inflammation, and inhibit tumor growth. Reishi mushroom supplements are available in various forms, including capsules, powders, extracts, and teas, and can be used to support cancer treatment and enhance overall well-being.

Astragalus (Astragalus membranaceus)

Astragalus is an adaptogenic herb widely used in TCM to support immune function, enhance vitality, and improve resilience to stress. Astragalus contains polysaccharides, flavonoids, saponins, and other bioactive compounds that modulate immune responses, reduce inflammation, and enhance cellular health. Astragalus has been studied for its potential to improve outcomes in cancer patients undergoing chemotherapy and radiation therapy by reducing treatment-related side effects, boosting immunity, and enhancing overall quality of life. Astragalus supplements are available in various forms, including capsules, extracts, and teas.

Ginger (Zingiber officinale)

Ginger is prized for its anti-inflammatory, anti-nausea, and digestive-supportive properties, making it particularly useful for cancer patients experiencing chemotherapy-induced nausea and vomiting. Ginger contains bioactive compounds such as gingerols and shogaols that help alleviate nausea, stimulate digestion, and reduce inflammation. Ginger can be consumed fresh, dried, or as a supplement, and incorporated into teas, soups, smoothies, and meals to support digestive health and reduce nausea during cancer treatment.

Conclusion

In conclusion, key herbs and plants such as turmeric, green tea, reishi mushroom, astragalus, and ginger have shown promise in supporting cancer treatment and symptom management. These herbs contain bioactive compounds with anti-inflammatory, antioxidant, immune-modulating, and anti-cancer properties that can complement conventional cancer therapies and improve overall quality of life for patients. Dr. Barbara integrates these key herbs and plants into her holistic approach to cancer care, selecting them based on their specific therapeutic actions and indications. As with any complementary therapy, it's essential for patients to consult with a qualified healthcare provider before incorporating herbs and plants into their cancer treatment regimen to ensure safety, appropriateness, and compatibility with existing treatment protocols.

CHAPTER SIX

Herbal Protocols for Different Types of Cancer

Herbal medicine offers a complementary approach to conventional cancer treatments, providing supportive care, symptom management, and potential anti-cancer effects for patients undergoing cancer treatment. Dr. Barbara tailors herbal protocols for different types of cancer based on the unique characteristics of each cancer, individual patient needs, treatment goals, and overall health status. While herbal protocols should be used as part of an integrative approach alongside conventional therapies, certain herbs have shown promise in supporting specific types of cancer. Here are some herbal protocols for different types of cancer:

Breast Cancer:

1. **Turmeric (Curcuma longa)**: Turmeric contains curcumin, a bioactive compound with potent anti-inflammatory and anti-cancer properties. Curcumin has been studied for its ability to inhibit breast cancer cell proliferation, induce apoptosis, and enhance the efficacy of conventional treatments such as chemotherapy and radiation therapy.

2. **Green Tea (Camellia sinensis)**: Green tea is rich in polyphenols, particularly epigallocatechin gallate (EGCG), which has been shown to inhibit breast cancer cell growth

and metastasis. Green tea consumption may also help reduce the risk of breast cancer recurrence and improve treatment outcomes.

3. **Flaxseed (Linum usitatissimum)**: Flaxseed is a rich source of lignans, omega-3 fatty acids, and fiber, which have been studied for their potential anti-cancer effects in breast cancer. Flaxseed consumption may help regulate hormone levels, reduce inflammation, and inhibit tumor growth in hormone-sensitive breast cancers.

Prostate Cancer:

1. **Saw Palmetto (Serenoa repens)**: Saw palmetto is commonly used to support prostate health and alleviate symptoms of benign prostatic hyperplasia (BPH). It contains bioactive compounds such as fatty acids and phytosterols that may help inhibit the growth of prostate cancer cells and reduce prostate-specific antigen (PSA) levels.

2. **Stinging Nettle (Urtica dioica)**: Stinging nettle root extract has been studied for its potential anti-inflammatory and anti-cancer effects in prostate cancer. It may help inhibit the growth of prostate cancer cells, reduce inflammation, and improve urinary symptoms associated with prostate enlargement.

3. **Pomegranate (Punica granatum)**: Pomegranate contains polyphenols, particularly ellagic acid and punicalagins, which have been shown to inhibit prostate cancer cell proliferation, induce apoptosis, and suppress tumor growth. Pomegranate juice or extract may help slow the progression of prostate cancer and improve treatment outcomes.

Colon Cancer:

1. **Aloe Vera (Aloe barbadensis)**: Aloe vera gel contains bioactive compounds such as polysaccharides, anthraquinones, and antioxidants that have been studied for their potential anti-cancer effects in colon cancer. Aloe vera may help inhibit tumor growth, reduce inflammation, and promote intestinal health.

2. **Ginger (Zingiber officinale)**: Ginger contains gingerols and shogaols, bioactive compounds with anti-inflammatory and anti-cancer properties. Ginger supplementation may help reduce colon cancer cell proliferation, inhibit tumor growth, and alleviate chemotherapy-induced nausea and vomiting.

3. **Turmeric (Curcuma longa)**: Turmeric and its active compound curcumin have been extensively studied for their anti-inflammatory and anti-cancer effects in colon cancer. Curcumin may help inhibit colon cancer cell proliferation, induce apoptosis, and enhance the efficacy of conventional treatments.

Lung Cancer:

1. **Ginseng (Panax ginseng)**: Ginseng contains ginsenosides, bioactive compounds with immune-modulating and anti-cancer properties. Ginseng supplementation may help enhance immune function, reduce inflammation, and improve quality of life in lung cancer patients undergoing treatment.

2. **Licorice Root (Glycyrrhiza glabra)**: Licorice root contains glycyrrhizin, a compound that has been studied for its potential anti-cancer effects in lung cancer. Licorice root may help inhibit lung cancer cell proliferation, induce apoptosis, and enhance the efficacy of chemotherapy and radiation therapy.

3. **Mullein (Verbascum thapsus)**: Mullein leaf and flower extracts have been traditionally used to support respiratory health and alleviate symptoms of cough and congestion. Mullein may help soothe irritated airways, reduce inflammation, and support lung function in lung cancer patients.

Conclusion

Herbal protocols for different types of cancer incorporate a variety of herbs and plants with potential anti-cancer, immune-modulating, and symptom-relieving properties. Dr. Barbara tailors herbal protocols to meet the specific needs of each patient, taking into account their cancer type, treatment regimen, overall health status, and individual preferences. While herbal medicine should be used as part of an integrative approach alongside conventional cancer treatments, certain herbs have shown promise in supporting cancer treatment and improving overall quality of life for patients. It's essential for patients to consult with a qualified healthcare provider knowledgeable in herbal medicine and integrative oncology to ensure safety, appropriateness, and compatibility with existing treatment protocols.

CHAPTER SEVEN

Integrating Herbal Therapies with Conventional Cancer Treatments

Integrative oncology, which combines conventional cancer treatments with complementary and alternative therapies such as herbal medicine, aims to optimize patient outcomes, improve quality of life, and reduce treatment-related side effects. Dr. Barbara recognizes the value of integrating herbal therapies with conventional cancer treatments, taking a holistic approach to care that addresses the physical, emotional, and spiritual aspects of healing. By combining the best of both worlds, patients can benefit from the synergistic effects of herbal therapies and conventional treatments while minimizing potential risks and maximizing therapeutic outcomes.

Collaborative Care and Communication

Integration of herbal therapies with conventional cancer treatments requires collaborative care and open communication between patients, oncologists, and healthcare providers. Dr. Barbara emphasizes the importance of building a multidisciplinary healthcare team that includes oncologists, naturopathic doctors, herbalists, nutritionists, and other healthcare professionals. This team-based approach ensures coordinated care, individualized treatment plans, and ongoing monitoring of patient progress throughout the cancer treatment journey.

Patients should inform their oncologists and healthcare providers about any herbal therapies, supplements, or dietary changes they are considering, as these may interact with conventional treatments or affect treatment outcomes. Open and honest communication enables healthcare providers to make informed decisions, tailor treatment plans to meet individual patient needs, and ensure safe and effective integration of herbal therapies with conventional cancer treatments.

Tailored Treatment Plans

Herbal therapies should be integrated into cancer treatment plans in a tailored and individualized manner, taking into account each patient's unique cancer diagnosis, treatment regimen, overall health status, and treatment goals. Dr. Barbara conducts thorough assessments and consultations to gain insight into patients' specific needs, preferences, and concerns, allowing her to develop customized treatment plans that combine the best of both conventional and herbal therapies.

Treatment plans may include a combination of conventional cancer treatments such as surgery, chemotherapy, radiation therapy, targeted therapy, and immunotherapy, alongside herbal therapies such as herbal remedies, dietary supplements, botanical extracts, and mind-body practices. Herbal therapies are selected based on their specific therapeutic properties, indications, and potential interactions with conventional treatments, ensuring compatibility and safety in the context of cancer care.

Monitoring and Evaluation

Regular monitoring and evaluation of patient progress are essential components of integrated cancer care, allowing healthcare providers to assess treatment efficacy, monitor for potential side effects or complications, and make adjustments to treatment plans as needed. Dr. Barbara collaborates closely with patients and their healthcare team to track treatment outcomes, evaluate symptom management, and address any concerns or challenges that may arise during the course of treatment.

Patients are encouraged to communicate openly with their healthcare providers about any changes in symptoms, treatment-related side effects, or concerns they may have throughout the cancer treatment process. This allows healthcare providers to provide timely support, guidance, and interventions to help patients manage symptoms, improve quality of life, and optimize treatment outcomes.

Education and Empowerment

Education and empowerment are integral components of integrated cancer care, empowering patients to make informed decisions about their treatment options, lifestyle choices, and self-care practices. Dr. Barbara provides patients with comprehensive education and resources about herbal therapies, conventional cancer treatments, dietary recommendations, lifestyle modifications, and supportive care strategies to help them navigate the complexities of cancer care and make empowered choices that align with their values and preferences.

Patients are encouraged to take an active role in their cancer treatment journey, ask questions, seek clarification, and advocate for their needs and preferences. By empowering patients with knowledge, skills, and resources, healthcare providers can help patients become active participants in their own care, improve treatment adherence and compliance, and enhance overall satisfaction and well-being throughout the cancer treatment process.

Conclusion

Integrating herbal therapies with conventional cancer treatments requires collaborative care, tailored treatment plans, regular monitoring and evaluation, and patient education and empowerment. By combining the best of both worlds, patients can benefit from the synergistic effects of herbal therapies and conventional treatments while minimizing potential risks and maximizing therapeutic outcomes. Dr. Barbara advocates for a holistic approach to cancer care that addresses the physical, emotional, and spiritual aspects of healing, empowering patients to make informed decisions about their treatment options and take an active role in their cancer treatment journey.

CHAPTER EIGHT

Addressing Side Effects and Complications of Cancer Treatment with Herbs

Cancer treatments such as chemotherapy, radiation therapy, surgery, and targeted therapy can often cause a range of side effects and complications that impact patients' quality of life and overall well-being. Herbal medicine offers a complementary approach to managing these side effects and complications, providing patients with natural and supportive care options that can alleviate symptoms, enhance treatment tolerance, and improve overall treatment outcomes. Dr. Barbara integrates herbs into her holistic approach to cancer care, selecting specific herbs based on their therapeutic properties and indications to address the unique needs of each patient.

Nausea and Vomiting:

1. **Ginger (Zingiber officinale)**: Ginger is well-known for its anti-nausea properties and can help alleviate chemotherapy-induced nausea and vomiting. Patients can consume ginger in various forms, including fresh ginger root, ginger tea, ginger capsules, or ginger candies, to help reduce nausea and improve digestive comfort.

2. **Peppermint (Mentha piperita)**: Peppermint has been traditionally used to soothe digestive discomfort and

alleviate nausea. Peppermint tea or peppermint oil capsules may help relieve chemotherapy-induced nausea and support gastrointestinal health during cancer treatment.

3. **Lemon Balm (Melissa officinalis)**: Lemon balm contains compounds that have mild sedative and anti-nausea effects, making it useful for managing chemotherapy-induced nausea and vomiting. Lemon balm tea or lemon balm supplements may help promote relaxation and reduce nausea symptoms.

Fatigue:

1. **Panax Ginseng (Panax ginseng)**: Panax ginseng is an adaptogenic herb that can help reduce cancer-related fatigue and improve energy levels. Ginseng supplements may help enhance physical endurance, reduce stress, and improve overall vitality in cancer patients undergoing treatment.

2. **Rhodiola (Rhodiola rosea)**: Rhodiola is another adaptogenic herb that can help alleviate fatigue, enhance mental clarity, and improve resilience to stress. Rhodiola supplements may help increase energy levels, reduce fatigue-related symptoms, and improve overall well-being during cancer treatment.

3. **Ashwagandha (Withaniasomnifera)**: Ashwagandha is an adaptogenic herb with rejuvenating and energizing properties. Ashwagandha supplements may help reduce fatigue, enhance physical performance, and support adrenal health in cancer patients undergoing treatment.

Pain and Inflammation:

1. **Turmeric (Curcuma longa)**: Turmeric contains curcumin, a potent anti-inflammatory compound that can help alleviate pain and inflammation associated with cancer treatment. Turmeric supplements or turmeric tea may help reduce pain, inflammation, and swelling, and improve overall comfort during cancer treatment.

2. **Devil's Claw (Harpagophytum procumbens)**: Devil's claw is a traditional herbal remedy for pain relief and inflammation. Devil's claw supplements may help alleviate chemotherapy-induced pain, joint discomfort, and inflammation, and improve mobility and quality of life.

3. **White Willow Bark (Salix alba)**: White willow bark contains salicin, a natural compound with analgesic and anti-inflammatory properties similar to aspirin. White willow bark supplements may help reduce cancer-related pain, headaches, and inflammation, and improve overall comfort during treatment.

Immune Support:

1. **Astragalus (Astragalus membranaceus)**: Astragalus is an immune-modulating herb that can help strengthen the immune system and enhance resilience to infections. Astragalus supplements may help support immune function, reduce the risk of infections, and improve overall well-being during cancer treatment.

2. **Echinacea (Echinacea purpurea)**: Echinacea is another immune-supportive herb that can help stimulate the body's natural defenses and enhance immune function. Echinacea supplements may help reduce the severity and duration of colds, flu, and other infections in cancer patients undergoing treatment.

3. **Medicinal Mushrooms (e.g., Reishi, Shiitake, Maitake)**: Medicinal mushrooms contain beta-glucans and other bioactive compounds that support immune function and enhance vitality. Mushroom supplements may help strengthen the immune system, reduce inflammation, and improve overall health and resilience during cancer treatment.

Digestive Support:

1. **Slippery Elm (Ulmus rubra)**: Slippery elm is a demulcent herb that can help soothe and protect the digestive tract.

Slippery elm supplements or teas may help alleviate chemotherapy-induced gastrointestinal symptoms such as nausea, heartburn, and diarrhea, and promote digestive comfort.

2. **Chamomile (Matricaria chamomilla)**: Chamomile is a gentle herb with anti-inflammatory and soothing properties that can help calm the digestive system and relieve gastrointestinal discomfort. Chamomile tea may help reduce chemotherapy-induced nausea, bloating, gas, and indigestion, and promote relaxation and digestive well-being.

3. **Fennel (Foeniculum vulgare)**: Fennel is a carminative herb that can help reduce gas, bloating, and digestive discomfort. Fennel tea or fennel supplements may help alleviate chemotherapy-induced gastrointestinal symptoms and support digestive health and comfort during cancer treatment.

Anxiety and Stress:

1. **Lavender (Lavandula angustifolia)**: Lavender is a calming herb with anxiolytic and sedative properties that can help reduce anxiety and promote relaxation. Lavender essential oil or lavender tea may help alleviate chemotherapy-related anxiety, stress, and insomnia, and improve overall emotional well-being.

2. **Passionflower (Passiflora incarnata)**: Passionflower is another calming herb with anxiolytic and sedative effects that can help reduce anxiety and improve sleep quality. Passionflower supplements or passionflower tea may help alleviate chemotherapy-induced anxiety, nervousness, and restlessness, and promote relaxation and emotional balance.

3. **Valerian (Valeriana officinalis)**: Valerian is a traditional herbal remedy for anxiety, stress, and insomnia. Valerian supplements or valerian tea may help reduce chemotherapy-related anxiety, tension, and sleep disturbances, and improve overall emotional well-being and quality of life.

Conclusion

In conclusion, herbal medicine offers a natural and supportive approach to managing the side effects and complications of cancer treatment, providing patients with safe, effective, and holistic care options that can alleviate symptoms, enhance treatment tolerance, and improve overall quality of life. Dr. Barbara integrates herbs into her comprehensive approach to cancer care, selecting specific herbs based on their therapeutic properties and indications to address the unique needs of each patient. By combining the best of both conventional and herbal therapies, patients can benefit from synergistic effects that optimize treatment outcomes and promote overall well-being throughout the cancer treatment journey.

CHAPTER NINE

Herbal Strategies for Cancer Prevention and Long-Term Wellness

Cancer prevention and long-term wellness are essential aspects of holistic health care that can be supported by incorporating herbal strategies into daily life. While herbal medicine should be used as part of a comprehensive approach to health that includes regular screenings, healthy lifestyle habits, and medical interventions when necessary, certain herbs have shown promise in supporting cancer prevention and promoting overall well-being. Dr. Barbara advocates for the integration of herbal strategies into daily routines to enhance immune function, reduce inflammation, and support cellular health, thereby reducing the risk of cancer and promoting long-term wellness.

Immune Support:

1. **Astragalus (Astragalus membranaceus)**: Astragalus is an adaptogenic herb that supports immune function and enhances resilience to stress. Regular use of astragalus supplements or teas can help strengthen the immune system, reduce the risk of infections, and promote overall well-being.

2. **Medicinal Mushrooms (e.g., Reishi, Shiitake, Maitake)**: Medicinal mushrooms contain beta-glucans and other

bioactive compounds that support immune function and enhance vitality. Incorporating mushroom supplements or mushroom extracts into the diet can help strengthen the immune system, reduce inflammation, and support long-term health.

3. **Echinacea (Echinacea purpurea)**: Echinacea is an immune-supportive herb that stimulates the body's natural defenses and enhances immune function. Taking echinacea supplements or drinking echinacea tea regularly can help reduce the risk of infections and support immune health.

Antioxidant Protection:

1. **Turmeric (Curcuma longa)**: Turmeric contains curcumin, a potent antioxidant with anti-inflammatory and anti-cancer properties. Adding turmeric to meals, teas, or smoothies can help reduce oxidative stress, inflammation, and cellular damage, thereby promoting long-term health and wellness.

2. **Green Tea (Camellia sinensis)**: Green tea is rich in polyphenols and catechins, powerful antioxidants that help protect cells from oxidative damage and reduce the risk of cancer. Drinking green tea regularly can support antioxidant defenses, promote cellular health, and enhance overall well-being.

3. **Berries (e.g., Blueberries, Strawberries, Raspberries)**: Berries are rich in vitamins, minerals, fiber, and antioxidants that help protect against oxidative stress and inflammation. Incorporating a variety of berries into the diet can support immune function, reduce the risk of chronic diseases, and promote long-term health.

Detoxification Support:

1. **Dandelion (Taraxacum officinale)**: Dandelion is a gentle detoxifying herb that supports liver health and promotes detoxification pathways in the body. Drinking dandelion tea or incorporating dandelion greens into salads can help support liver function, improve digestion, and enhance overall detoxification.

2. **Milk Thistle (Silybum marianum)**: Milk thistle contains silymarin, a compound with antioxidant and hepatoprotective properties that supports liver health and detoxification. Taking milk thistle supplements or drinking milk thistle tea can help protect the liver from toxins and promote overall well-being.

3. **Cilantro (Coriandrum sativum)**: Cilantro is a natural chelating agent that helps remove heavy metals and toxins from the body. Adding fresh cilantro to salads, soups, or smoothies can support detoxification, improve digestion, and promote long-term wellness.

Stress Management:

1. **Ashwagandha (Withaniasomnifera)**: Ashwagandha is an adaptogenic herb that helps the body adapt to stress, regulate cortisol levels, and promote relaxation. Taking ashwagandha supplements or drinking ashwagandha tea can help reduce stress, improve sleep quality, and support overall well-being.

2. **Holy Basil (Ocimum sanctum)**: Holy basil, also known as Tulsi, is a calming herb with adaptogenic properties that helps reduce stress and promote mental clarity. Drinking holy basil tea or taking holy basil supplements can help alleviate stress, improve cognitive function, and enhance overall resilience to stress.

3. **Lemon Balm (Melissa officinalis)**: Lemon balm is a soothing herb with mild sedative properties that helps calm the nervous system and promote relaxation. Drinking lemon balm tea or taking lemon balm supplements can help reduce stress, anxiety, and tension, and promote overall emotional well-being.

Conclusion

In conclusion, herbal strategies play a valuable role in cancer prevention and long-term wellness by supporting immune function, reducing oxidative stress and inflammation, promoting detoxification, and enhancing stress management. Dr. Barbara advocates for the integration of herbal strategies into daily routines to promote overall health and well-being, reduce the risk of cancer, and support long-term vitality. By incorporating immune-supportive herbs, antioxidant-rich foods, detoxifying herbs, and stress-reducing herbs into daily life, individuals can optimize their health and reduce the risk of chronic diseases, including cancer, promoting a lifetime of wellness.

Chaparral:

Definition: Chaparral, scientifically known as Larrea tridentata, is a shrub native to the southwestern United States and northern Mexico. It has been used for centuries by Native American tribes for its medicinal properties and is commonly used in herbal medicine today.

Ingredients: Chaparral contains several bioactive compounds, including nordihydroguaiaretic acid (NDGA), flavonoids, lignans, and volatile oils. NDGA is believed to be the primary active compound responsible for many of chaparral's therapeutic effects.

How to Prepare: Chaparral can be prepared and consumed in various forms, including teas, tinctures, capsules, and topical preparations. To make tea, dried chaparral leaves are steeped in hot water for several minutes before being strained and consumed. Tinctures are prepared by steeping the herb in alcohol or vinegar to extract its active compounds.

Dosage: The appropriate dosage of chaparral can vary depending on the specific form and intended use. It's important to follow the recommended dosage on the product label or consult with a healthcare professional for personalized guidance.

How to Use: Chaparral tea or tincture is typically taken orally. It can also be applied topically to the skin for certain conditions. It's important to use chaparral products as directed and to discontinue use if any adverse effects occur.

Side Effects: Chaparral is generally considered safe for most people when used in moderate amounts. However, excessive intake or prolonged use may lead to liver toxicity or other adverse effects. It may also interact with certain medications or have adverse effects in individuals with certain health conditions. It's important to use chaparral under the guidance of a healthcare professional and to discontinue use if any adverse effects occur.

Cocolmeca:

Definition: Cocolmeca, also known as Smilax ornata or sarsaparilla, is a flowering vine native to Mexico and Central America. It has been used traditionally in Mexican and Central American folk medicine for its purported medicinal properties.

Ingredients: Cocolmeca contains various bioactive compounds, including saponins, flavonoids, and plant sterols. These compounds are believed to contribute to the herb's medicinal properties, including its potential as a diuretic, blood purifier, and anti-inflammatory agent.

How to Prepare: Cocolmeca is commonly prepared and consumed as an herbal tea or decoction. To make tea, dried cocolmeca roots or leaves are steeped in hot water for several minutes before being strained and consumed. Decoctions involve boiling the roots or leaves in water to extract their active compounds.

Dosage: The appropriate dosage of cocolmeca can vary depending on factors such as age, health status, and the specific preparation being used. It's important to follow the recommended dosage on the product label or consult with a qualified herbalist or healthcare professional for personalized guidance.

How to Use: Cocolmeca tea or decoction is typically taken orally. It can also be used topically for certain skin conditions. It's important to use cocolmeca products as directed and to discontinue use if any adverse effects occur.

Side Effects: Cocolmeca is generally considered safe for most people when used in moderate amounts. However, excessive intake may lead to digestive upset or other adverse effects. It may also interact with certain medications or have adverse effects in individuals with certain health conditions. It's important to use cocolmeca under the guidance of a healthcare professional and to discontinue use if any adverse effects occur.

Contribo:

Definition: Contribo, also known as Aristolochiatrilobata, is a vine native to the Caribbean and Central America. It has been used traditionally in folk medicine for various purposes, including as a remedy for digestive issues, inflammation, and pain relief.

Ingredients: Contribo contains several bioactive compounds, including aristolochic acids, flavonoids, and alkaloids. These compounds are believed to contribute to the herb's medicinal properties, including its potential as an anti-inflammatory and analgesic agent.

How to Prepare: Contribo is typically prepared and consumed as an herbal tea or decoction. To make tea, dried contribo leaves or stems are steeped in hot water for several minutes before being strained and consumed. Decoctions involve boiling the leaves or stems in water to extract their active compounds.

Dosage: The appropriate dosage of contribo can vary depending on factors such as age, health status, and the specific preparation being used. It's important to follow the recommended dosage on the product label or consult with a qualified herbalist or healthcare professional for personalized guidance.

How to Use: Contribo tea or decoction is typically taken orally. It's important to use contribo products as directed and to discontinue use if any adverse effects occur.

Side Effects: Contribo contains aristolochic acids, which have been associated with serious adverse effects, including kidney damage and cancer. Due to these safety concerns, the use of contribo is highly discouraged, and it's important to avoid products containing aristolochic acids. Individuals should seek alternative remedies for their health needs.

Dandelion Root:

Definition: Dandelion, scientifically known as Taraxacum officinale, is a common flowering plant found worldwide. While often considered a pesky weed, dandelion has a long history of use in traditional medicine for its various health benefits.

Ingredients: Dandelion root contains several bioactive compounds, including sesquiterpene lactones, triterpenes, flavonoids, and polysaccharides. These compounds are believed to contribute to the herb's medicinal properties, including its potential as a diuretic, digestive aid, and liver tonic.

How to Prepare: Dandelion root can be prepared and consumed in various forms, including teas, tinctures, capsules, and extracts. To make tea, dried dandelion root is steeped in hot water for several minutes before being strained and consumed. Tinctures are prepared by steeping the root in alcohol or vinegar to extract its active compounds.

Dosage: The appropriate dosage of dandelion root can vary depending on factors such as age, health status, and the specific preparation being used. It's important to follow the recommended dosage on the product label or consult with a qualified herbalist or healthcare professional for personalized guidance.

How to Use: Dandelion root tea, tincture, or capsules are typically taken orally. It's important to use dandelion root products as directed and to discontinue use if any adverse effects occur.

Side Effects: Dandelion root is generally considered safe for most people when used in moderate amounts. However, some individuals may experience allergic reactions or digestive upset. It may also interact with certain medications or have adverse effects in individuals with certain health conditions. It's important to use dandelion root under the guidance of a healthcare professional and to discontinue use if any adverse effects occur.

Green Food Plus:

Definition: Green Food Plus is a dietary supplement formulated to provide a concentrated source of nutrients derived from various green plants. It's designed to support overall health and well-being by delivering essential vitamins, minerals, antioxidants, and phytonutrients.

Ingredients: Green Food Plus typically contains a blend of powdered green vegetables, grasses, algae, and other plant-based ingredients. Common ingredients may include wheatgrass, barley grass, spirulina, chlorella, alfalfa, kale, spinach, and broccoli, among others.

How to Prepare: Green Food Plus is usually available in powder form and can be mixed with water, juice, or smoothies. It's important to follow the recommended dosage on the product label and to consume it as part of a balanced diet.

Dosage: The appropriate dosage of Green Food Plus can vary depending on the specific product and individual needs. It's important to follow the recommended dosage on the product label or consult with a healthcare professional for personalized guidance.

How to Use: Green Food Plus powder is typically mixed with water, juice, or smoothies and consumed orally. It's often taken once or twice daily, preferably with meals, to maximize nutrient absorption.

Side Effects: Green Food Plus is generally considered safe for most people when used as directed. However, some individuals may experience digestive upset or allergic reactions to certain ingredients. It's important to consult with a healthcare provider before starting any new supplement regimen, especially if you have underlying health conditions or are taking medications.

Guaco:

Definition: Guaco, also known as Mikania cordata or Mikania glomerata, is a medicinal plant native to Central and South America. It has a long history of use in traditional medicine for its potential therapeutic properties.

Ingredients: Guaco contains several bioactive compounds, including coumarins, flavonoids, tannins, and saponins. These compounds are believed to contribute to the herb's medicinal properties, including its potential as an expectorant, anti-inflammatory, and antispasmodic agent.

How to Prepare: Guaco is typically prepared and consumed as an herbal tea or infusion. To make tea, dried guaco leaves are steeped in hot water for several minutes before being strained and consumed.

Dosage: The appropriate dosage of guaco can vary depending on factors such as age, health status, and the specific preparation being used. It's important to follow the recommended dosage on the product label or consult with a qualified herbalist or healthcare professional for personalized guidance.

How to Use: Guaco tea is typically taken orally. It can be consumed on its own or mixed with honey or other herbal teas for added flavor.

Side Effects: Guaco is generally considered safe for most people when used in moderate amounts. However, some individuals may experience allergic reactions or digestive upset. It may also interact with certain medications or have adverse effects in individuals with certain health conditions. It's important to use guaco under the guidance of a healthcare professional and to discontinue use if any adverse effects occur.

Herban Iron:

Definition: Herban Iron is a dietary supplement designed to provide an easily absorbable form of iron to support healthy iron levels in the body. It's particularly beneficial for individuals with iron deficiency or anemia.

Ingredients: Herban Iron typically contains iron in the form of ferrous bisglycinate, which is a highly bioavailable and gentle form of iron that is less likely to cause digestive upset or constipation compared to other forms of iron. It may also contain other ingredients such as vitamin C to enhance iron absorption.

How to Prepare: Herban Iron is usually available in capsule or liquid form. Capsules are taken orally with water, while liquid forms may be mixed with water or juice before consumption. It's important to follow the recommended dosage on the product label.

Dosage: The appropriate dosage of Herban Iron depends on factors such as age, gender, and the severity of iron deficiency. It's important to consult with a healthcare professional to determine the correct dosage for individual needs.

How to Use: Herban Iron capsules are typically taken orally with water, while liquid forms may be mixed with water or juice before consumption. It's important to take Herban Iron as directed and to avoid taking it with dairy products, antacids, or other substances that may interfere with iron absorption.

Side Effects: While Herban Iron is generally considered safe for most people when used as directed, some individuals may experience mild side effects such as gastrointestinal discomfort or constipation. It's important to consult with a healthcare professional before starting any new supplement regimen, especially if you have underlying health conditions or are taking medications.

Hydrangea:

Definition: Hydrangea, scientifically known as Hydrangea arborescens, is a flowering shrub native to North America. It has been used traditionally in herbal medicine for its potential diuretic and anti-inflammatory properties.

Ingredients: Hydrangea contains several bioactive compounds, including saponins, flavonoids, and glycosides. These compounds are believed to contribute to the herb's medicinal properties, including its potential as a diuretic, kidney tonic, and anti-inflammatory agent.

How to Prepare: Hydrangea root is typically prepared and consumed as an herbal tea or tincture. To make tea, dried hydrangea root is steeped in hot water for several minutes before being strained and consumed. Tinctures are prepared by steeping the root in alcohol or vinegar to extract its active compounds.

Dosage: The appropriate dosage of hydrangea can vary depending on factors such as age, health status, and the specific preparation being used. It's important to follow the recommended dosage on the product label or consult with a qualified herbalist or healthcare professional for personalized guidance.

How to Use: Hydrangea tea or tincture is typically taken orally. It's important to use hydrangea products as directed and to discontinue use if any adverse effects occur.

Side Effects: Hydrangea is generally considered safe for most people when used in moderate amounts. However, some individuals may experience digestive upset or allergic reactions. It may also interact with certain medications or have adverse effects in individuals with certain health conditions. It's important to use hydrangea under the guidance of a healthcare professional and to discontinue use if any adverse effects occur.

Irish Moss:

Definition: Irish Moss, scientifically known as Chondrus crispus, is a species of red algae or seaweed native to the Atlantic coastlines of Europe and North America. It has been used for centuries in traditional Irish and Scottish cuisine, as well as in herbal medicine.

Ingredients: Irish Moss is rich in various nutrients, including iodine, sulfur compounds, vitamins (such as vitamin A, vitamin K, and vitamin B12), minerals (including calcium, magnesium, potassium, and sodium), and polysaccharides (such as carrageenan). These nutrients are believed to contribute to the herb's potential health benefits.

How to Prepare: Irish Moss is typically prepared by soaking it in water to rehydrate and soften it before use. It can be added to soups, stews, smoothies, desserts, and other dishes as a thickening agent or nutritional supplement.

Dosage: The appropriate dosage of Irish Moss can vary depending on factors such as age, health status, and the specific preparation being used. It's important to follow recipes or guidelines for culinary use and to consult with a healthcare professional for guidance on using Irish Moss as a dietary supplement.

How to Use: Irish Moss can be used in culinary applications to add thickness and nutritional value to dishes. It can also be consumed as a dietary supplement in the form of capsules, powders, or extracts.

Side Effects: Irish Moss is generally considered safe for most people when consumed in moderate amounts as part of a balanced diet. However, some individuals may be allergic to seaweed or carrageenan, a compound found in Irish Moss that is used as a food additive. It's important to discontinue use if any adverse effects occur and to consult with a healthcare professional if you have any concerns.

Irish Sea Moss:

Definition: Irish Sea Moss is a term often used interchangeably with Irish Moss, referring to the same species of red algae, Chondrus crispus. It's harvested from the rocky shores of the Atlantic coastlines of Europe and North America.

Ingredients: Irish Sea Moss shares the same nutritional profile as Irish Moss, containing iodine, vitamins, minerals, and polysaccharides. It's valued for its potential health benefits, including supporting thyroid function, boosting immune health, and promoting digestion.

How to Prepare: Irish Sea Moss is prepared in the same way as Irish Moss, by soaking it in water to rehydrate and soften it before use. It can be used in culinary applications or consumed as a dietary supplement.

Dosage: The dosage of Irish Sea Moss depends on the form and intended use. As a dietary supplement, it's important to follow the recommended dosage on the product label or consult with a healthcare professional for personalized guidance.

How to Use: Irish Sea Moss can be used in various culinary applications, including soups, smoothies, desserts, and sauces. It can also be consumed as a dietary supplement in the form of capsules, powders, or extracts.

Side Effects: Similar to Irish Moss, Irish Sea Moss is generally considered safe for most people when consumed in moderate amounts. However, individuals with seaweed allergies or sensitivities to carrageenan should exercise caution. It's important to discontinue use if any adverse effects occur and to consult with a healthcare professional if you have any concerns.

Lymphalin:

Definition: Lymphalin is a herbal supplement formulated to support lymphatic system health. The lymphatic system plays a crucial role in immune function and waste removal in the body, and Lymphalin is designed to promote its proper function.

Ingredients: Lymphalin typically contains a blend of herbs and botanical extracts known for their traditional use in supporting lymphatic system health. Common ingredients may include cleavers, red clover, echinacea, burdock root, and calendula, among others.

How to Prepare: Lymphalin is usually available in capsule or liquid form. Capsules are taken orally with water, while liquid forms may be mixed with water or juice before consumption. It's important to follow the recommended dosage on the product label.

Dosage: The appropriate dosage of Lymphalin can vary depending on the specific product and individual needs. It's important to follow the recommended dosage on the product label or consult with a healthcare professional for personalized guidance.

How to Use: Lymphalin capsules are typically taken orally with water, while liquid forms may be mixed with water or juice before consumption. It's often recommended to take Lymphalin on an empty stomach for optimal absorption.

Side Effects: Lymphalin is generally considered safe for most people when used as directed. However, some individuals may experience mild side effects such as gastrointestinal discomfort or allergic reactions to certain ingredients. It's important to consult with a healthcare provider before starting any new supplement regimen, especially if you have underlying health conditions or are taking medications.

Manjakani:

Definition: Manjakani, also known as Quercus infectoria or oak gall, is a natural substance derived from the oak tree. It has been used for centuries in traditional medicine for its potential health benefits, particularly for women's health and vaginal tightening.

Ingredients: Manjakani contains various bioactive compounds, including tannins, flavonoids, and gallic acid. These compounds are believed to contribute to the herb's medicinal properties, including its potential as an astringent and antiseptic agent.

How to Prepare: Manjakani is typically available in powder, capsule, or liquid extract form. It can be taken orally or used topically depending on the intended use. For vaginal tightening, manjakani may be applied topically as a gel or inserted into the vagina in capsule form.

Dosage: The appropriate dosage of manjakani can vary depending on factors such as age, health status, and the specific preparation being used. It's important to follow the recommended dosage on the product label or consult with a qualified herbalist or healthcare professional for personalized guidance.

How to Use: Manjakani can be taken orally or used topically depending on the intended use. It's important to use manjakani products as directed and to discontinue use if any adverse effects occur.

Side Effects: Manjakani is generally considered safe for most people when used in moderate amounts. However, some individuals may experience allergic reactions or skin irritation when used topically. It's important to use manjakani under the guidance of a healthcare professional and to discontinue use if any adverse effects occur.

Red Clover:

Definition: Red clover, scientifically known as Trifolium pratense, is a flowering plant belonging to the legume family. It's native to Europe, Western Asia, and Northwest Africa but has been naturalized in many other regions. Red clover has been used in traditional medicine for various purposes, including its potential to support women's health and menopausal symptoms.

Ingredients: Red clover contains several bioactive compounds, including isoflavones (such as genistein and daidzein), flavonoids, and phytoestrogens. These compounds are believed to contribute to the herb's medicinal properties, including its potential as a hormone-balancing agent and its ability to support cardiovascular health.

How to Prepare: Red clover is typically prepared and consumed as an herbal tea or tincture. To make tea, dried red clover flowers are steeped in hot water for several minutes before being strained and consumed. Tinctures are prepared by steeping the flowers in alcohol or vinegar to extract their active compounds.

Dosage: The appropriate dosage of red clover can vary depending on factors such as age, health status, and the specific preparation being used. It's important to follow the recommended dosage on the product label or consult with a qualified herbalist or healthcare professional for personalized guidance.

How to Use: Red clover tea or tincture is typically taken orally. It's important to use red clover products as directed and to discontinue use if any adverse effects occur.

Side Effects: Red clover is generally considered safe for most people when used in moderate amounts. However, some individuals may experience allergic reactions or digestive upset. It may also interact with certain medications or have adverse effects in individuals with certain health conditions. It's important to use red clover under the guidance of a healthcare professional and to discontinue use if any adverse effects occur.

Red Raspberry:

Definition: Red raspberry, scientifically known as Rubus idaeus, is a species of raspberry native to Europe and northern Asia. It's widely cultivated for its delicious berries and has been used in traditional medicine for various purposes, including its potential to support women's health during pregnancy and childbirth.

Ingredients: Red raspberry contains several bioactive compounds, including flavonoids, ellagic acid, anthocyanins, and vitamin C. These compounds are believed to contribute to the herb's medicinal properties, including its potential as an antioxidant, anti-inflammatory, and uterine tonic.

How to Prepare: Red raspberry leaf is typically prepared and consumed as an herbal tea or infusion. To make tea, dried red raspberry leaves are steeped in hot water for several minutes before being strained and consumed.

Dosage: The appropriate dosage of red raspberry leaf can vary depending on factors such as age, health status, and the specific preparation being used. It's important to follow the recommended dosage on the product label or consult with a qualified herbalist or healthcare professional for personalized guidance.

How to Use: Red raspberry leaf tea is typically taken orally. It's often recommended for pregnant individuals in the later stages of pregnancy to support uterine health and prepare for childbirth. It's important to use red raspberry leaf products as directed and to discontinue use if any adverse effects occur.

Side Effects: Red raspberry leaf is generally considered safe for most people when used in moderate amounts. However, some individuals may experience allergic reactions or digestive upset. Pregnant individuals should consult with a healthcare professional before using red raspberry leaf, especially if they have any underlying health conditions or are taking medications. It's important to use red raspberry leaf under the guidance of a healthcare professional and to discontinue use if any adverse effects occur.

Rhubarb:

Definition: Rhubarb, scientifically known as Rheum rhabarbarum, is a perennial plant cultivated for its edible stalks. While primarily used in culinary applications, rhubarb has also been utilized in traditional medicine for its potential health benefits, particularly for digestive health.

Ingredients: Rhubarb stalks contain various bioactive compounds, including anthraquinones (such as emodin and rhein), fiber, vitamins (such as vitamin K), and minerals (including calcium and potassium). These compounds are believed to contribute to the herb's medicinal properties, including its potential as a laxative and digestive aid.

How to Prepare: Rhubarb stalks are typically cooked before consumption, as the raw stalks are very tart and can be unpleasant to eat. They are often used in pies, crisps, jams, sauces, and other desserts, as well as in savory dishes. Rhubarb can also be used to make compotes, jams, and preserves.

Dosage: There is no specific dosage for rhubarb in culinary applications, as it is used as a food rather than a medicinal herb. However, when used for its potential laxative effects, it's important to consume rhubarb in moderation to avoid gastrointestinal upset.

How to Use: Rhubarb stalks can be chopped and cooked in various dishes, including pies, sauces, and jams. It's important to remove and discard the leaves, as they contain toxic compounds. When using rhubarb for its potential laxative effects, it's typically consumed as part of a cooked dish or in the form of a rhubarb-based herbal remedy.

Side Effects: Rhubarb stalks are generally safe for most people when consumed in moderate amounts as part of a balanced diet. However, excessive intake may lead to digestive upset or adverse effects due to the presence of oxalic acid, which can bind to calcium and form kidney stones in susceptible individuals. It's important to use rhubarb in moderation and to consult with a healthcare professional if you have any concerns or underlying health conditions.

Sarsaparilla:

Definition: Sarsaparilla refers to several species of plants belonging to the Smilax genus, including Smilax regelii and Smilax officinalis. It has been used historically in traditional medicine for its potential health benefits, particularly for its purported detoxifying and anti-inflammatory properties.

Ingredients: Sarsaparilla contains various bioactive compounds, including saponins (such as sarsaponin and smilagenin), flavonoids, phenolic acids, and sterols. These compounds are believed to contribute to the herb's medicinal properties, including its potential as a diuretic, blood purifier, and anti-inflammatory agent.

How to Prepare: Sarsaparilla root is typically prepared and consumed as an herbal tea, decoction, or tincture. To make tea, dried sarsaparilla root is steeped in hot water for several minutes before being strained and consumed. Decoctions involve boiling the root in water to extract its active compounds, while tinctures are prepared by steeping the root in alcohol or vinegar.

Dosage: The appropriate dosage of sarsaparilla can vary depending on factors such as age, health status, and the specific preparation being used. It's important to follow the recommended dosage on the product label or consult with a qualified herbalist or healthcare professional for personalized guidance.

How to Use: Sarsaparilla tea or tincture is typically taken orally. It's important to use sarsaparilla products as directed and to discontinue use if any adverse effects occur.

Side Effects: Sarsaparilla is generally considered safe for most people when used in moderate amounts. However, some individuals may experience allergic reactions or digestive upset. It may also interact with certain medications or have adverse effects in individuals with certain health conditions. It's important to use sarsaparilla under the guidance of a healthcare professional and to discontinue use if any adverse effects occur.

Valerian:

Definition: Valerian, scientifically known as Valeriana officinalis, is a perennial flowering plant native to Europe and Asia. It has been used for centuries in traditional medicine for its potential calming and sedative effects.

Ingredients: Valerian root contains several bioactive compounds, including valerenic acid, valepotriates, and volatile oils. These compounds are believed to contribute to the herb's medicinal properties, including its potential as a sedative, anxiolytic, and sleep aid.

How to Prepare: Valerian root is typically prepared and consumed as an herbal tea, tincture, or capsule. To make tea, dried valerian root is steeped in hot water for several minutes before being strained and consumed. Tinctures are prepared by steeping the root in alcohol or vinegar to extract its active compounds.

Dosage: The appropriate dosage of valerian can vary depending on factors such as age, health status, and the specific preparation being used. It's important to follow the recommended dosage on the product label or consult with a qualified herbalist or healthcare professional for personalized guidance.

How to Use: Valerian tea, tincture, or capsules are typically taken orally. It's often consumed in the evening as a sleep aid or during times of stress or anxiety. It's important to use valerian products as directed and to discontinue use if any adverse effects occur.

Side Effects: Valerian is generally considered safe for most people when used in moderate amounts. However, some individuals may experience mild side effects such as drowsiness, headache, or gastrointestinal upset. It may also interact with certain medications or have adverse effects in individuals with certain health conditions. It's important to use valerian under the guidance of a healthcare professional and to discontinue use if any adverse effects occur.

Wild Cherry Bark:

Definition: Wild cherry bark, scientifically known as Prunus serotina, is the bark obtained from the black cherry tree native to North America. It has been used traditionally in Native American and folk medicine for its potential health benefits, particularly for respiratory and digestive issues.

Ingredients: Wild cherry bark contains various bioactive compounds, including cyanogenic glycosides (such as prunasin and amygdalin), flavonoids, and phenolic acids. These compounds are believed to contribute to the herb's medicinal properties, including its potential as an expectorant, cough suppressant, and mild sedative.

How to Prepare: Wild cherry bark is typically prepared and consumed as an herbal tea, decoction, or syrup. To make tea, dried wild cherry bark is steeped in hot water for several minutes before being strained and consumed. Decoctions involve boiling the bark in water to extract its active compounds, while syrups are made by simmering the bark with sugar or honey to create a thick, sweet liquid.

Dosage: The appropriate dosage of wild cherry bark can vary depending on factors such as age, health status, and the specific preparation being used. It's important to follow the recommended dosage on the product label or consult with a qualified herbalist or healthcare professional for personalized guidance.

How to Use: Wild cherry bark tea, decoction, or syrup is typically taken orally. It's often consumed to soothe coughs, sore throats, and other respiratory symptoms. It's important to use wild cherry bark products as directed and to discontinue use if any adverse effects occur.

Side Effects: Wild cherry bark is generally considered safe for most people when used in moderate amounts. However, it contains cyanogenic glycosides, which can release cyanide in the body when metabolized. While the risk of cyanide poisoning from consuming wild cherry bark is low when used appropriately, excessive intake or prolonged use may lead to adverse effects. It's important to use wild cherry bark under the guidance of a healthcare professional and to discontinue use if any adverse effects occur.

Yellowdock:

Definition: Yellowdock, scientifically known as Rumex crispus, is a perennial flowering plant native to Europe and western Asia but is also found in North America. It has a long history of use in traditional medicine, particularly among Indigenous peoples, for its potential health benefits.

Ingredients: Yellowdock root contains various bioactive compounds, including anthraquinone glycosides (such as emodin and chrysophanol), tannins, and vitamins (including vitamin A and vitamin C). These compounds are believed to contribute to the herb's medicinal properties, including its potential as a laxative, blood cleanser, and liver tonic.

How to Prepare: Yellowdock root is typically prepared and consumed as an herbal tea, tincture, or capsule. To make tea, dried yellowdock root is steeped in hot water for several minutes before being strained and consumed. Tinctures are prepared by steeping the root in alcohol or vinegar to extract its active compounds.

Dosage: The appropriate dosage of yellowdock can vary depending on factors such as age, health status, and the specific preparation being used. It's important to follow the recommended dosage on the product label or consult with a qualified herbalist or healthcare professional for personalized guidance.

How to Use: Yellowdock tea, tincture, or capsules are typically taken orally. It's often consumed to support digestion, promote bowel regularity, and cleanse the blood. It's important to use yellowdock products as directed and to discontinue use if any adverse effects occur.

Side Effects: Yellowdock is generally considered safe for most people when used in moderate amounts. However, some individuals may experience mild side effects such as gastrointestinal upset or allergic reactions. It may also interact with certain medications or have adverse effects in individuals with certain health conditions. It's important to use yellowdock under the guidance of a healthcare professional and to discontinue use if any adverse effects occur.

Yellowdock Root:

Definition: Yellowdock root, scientifically known as Rumex crispus, is the root of a perennial flowering plant native to Europe and western Asia, also found in North America. It has a long history of use in traditional medicine, particularly among Indigenous peoples, for its potential health benefits.

Ingredients: Yellowdock root contains various bioactive compounds, including anthraquinone glycosides (such as emodin and chrysophanol), tannins, and vitamins (including vitamin A and vitamin C). These compounds are believed to contribute to the herb's medicinal properties, including its potential as a laxative, blood cleanser, and liver tonic.

How to Prepare: Yellowdock root is typically prepared and consumed as an herbal tea, tincture, or capsule. To make tea, dried yellowdock root is steeped in hot water for several minutes before being strained and consumed. Tinctures are prepared by steeping the root in alcohol or vinegar to extract its active compounds.

Dosage: The appropriate dosage of yellowdock root can vary depending on factors such as age, health status, and the specific preparation being used. It's important to follow the recommended dosage on the product label or consult with a qualified herbalist or healthcare professional for personalized guidance.

How to Use: Yellowdock root tea, tincture, or capsules are typically taken orally. It's often consumed to support digestion, promote bowel regularity, and cleanse the blood. It's important to use yellowdock root products as directed and to discontinue use if any adverse effects occur.

Side Effects: Yellowdock root is generally considered safe for most people when used in moderate amounts. However, some individuals may experience mild side effects such as gastrointestinal upset or allergic reactions. It may also interact with certain medications or have adverse effects in individuals with certain health conditions. It's important to use yellowdock root under the guidance of a healthcare professional and to discontinue use if any adverse effects occur.

Agrimony:

Definition: Agrimony, scientifically known as Agrimonia eupatoria, is a perennial herbaceous plant native to Europe, Asia, and North America. It has a long history of use in traditional medicine, particularly in European folk medicine, for its potential health benefits.

Ingredients: Agrimony contains various bioactive compounds, including tannins, flavonoids, phenolic acids, and volatile oils. These compounds are believed to contribute to the herb's medicinal properties, including its potential as an astringent, anti-inflammatory, and digestive aid.

How to Prepare: Agrimony is typically prepared and consumed as an herbal tea, tincture, or poultice. To make tea, dried agrimony leaves and flowers are steeped in hot water for several minutes before being strained and consumed. Tinctures are prepared by steeping the herb in alcohol or vinegar to extract its active compounds.

Dosage: The appropriate dosage of agrimony can vary depending on factors such as age, health status, and the specific preparation being used. It's important to follow the recommended dosage on the product label or consult with a qualified herbalist or healthcare professional for personalized guidance.

How to Use: Agrimony tea, tincture, or poultice is typically taken orally or applied topically. It's often consumed to soothe gastrointestinal issues, such as indigestion and diarrhea, or used externally to treat skin conditions.

Side Effects: Agrimony is generally considered safe for most people when used in moderate amounts. However, some individuals may experience allergic reactions or gastrointestinal upset. It may also interact with certain medications or have adverse effects in individuals with certain health conditions. It's important to use agrimony under the guidance of a healthcare professional and to discontinue use if any adverse effects occur.

Tila:

Definition: Tila, also known as linden flower or lime blossom, refers to the flowers of the Tilia genus, primarily Tilia europaea and Tilia cordata. These trees are native to Europe, but they are also cultivated in other regions for their fragrant and medicinal flowers.

Ingredients: Tila flowers contain various bioactive compounds, including flavonoids, phenolic acids, and volatile oils. These compounds are believed to contribute to the herb's medicinal properties, including its potential as a mild sedative, anxiolytic, and anti-inflammatory agent.

How to Prepare: Tila flowers are typically prepared and consumed as an herbal tea or infusion. To make tea, dried tila flowers are steeped in hot water for several minutes before being strained and consumed.

Dosage: The appropriate dosage of tila can vary depending on factors such as age, health status, and the specific preparation being used. It's important to follow the recommended dosage on the product label or consult with a qualified herbalist or healthcare professional for personalized guidance.

How to Use: Tila tea is typically taken orally. It's often consumed in the evening as a calming bedtime beverage or during times of stress or anxiety. It's important to use tila products as directed and to discontinue use if any adverse effects occur.

Side Effects: Tila is generally considered safe for most people when used in moderate amounts. However, some individuals may experience allergic reactions or digestive upset. It may also interact with certain medications or have adverse effects in individuals with certain health conditions. It's important to use tila under the guidance of a healthcare professional and to discontinue use if any adverse effects occur.

Cell Food:

Definition: Cell Food is a dietary supplement marketed as a highly oxygenating and alkalizing formula. It's claimed to support overall health and vitality by providing essential nutrients and oxygen to the cells.

Ingredients: The exact ingredients of Cell Food can vary depending on the brand, but it typically contains a proprietary blend of minerals, enzymes, electrolytes, and trace elements. Some common ingredients may include purified water, dissolved oxygen, seawater extract, and plant-based enzymes.

How to Prepare: Cell Food is usually available in liquid form and is typically taken orally. It can be consumed directly or diluted in water or juice before consumption.

Dosage: The dosage of Cell Food can vary depending on the specific product and individual needs. It's important to follow the recommended dosage on the product label or consult with a healthcare professional for personalized guidance.

How to Use: Cell Food is typically taken orally, either directly or mixed into water or juice. It's important to shake the bottle well before use and to store it according to the manufacturer's instructions.

Side Effects: Cell Food is generally considered safe for most people when used as directed. However, some individuals may experience mild digestive upset or allergic reactions to certain ingredients. It's essential to consult with a healthcare provider before starting any new supplement regimen, especially if you have underlying health conditions or are taking medications.

THE END